Table of Contents

INTRODUCTION

Inflammation is our body's first response to injury and disease. Over time, inflammation can harm the body and may cause disease. Smoking as well as poor exercise, sleep and eating habits can increase risk of inflammation. You can make healthy choices to reduce inflammation in your body by changing your lifestyle and maintaining good eating habits. A lot inflammatory conditions nowadays are basically cause by unhealthy eating habits and sedentary lifestyle, we tend to eat inorganic foods like junks because they are readily available for consumption whereas they cause a lot of damage in the body. An individual is said to be the product of what he or she eats.

Symptoms of Chronic Inflammation

The following are the symptoms the body system shows in case of inflammation of any kind. These symptoms are often neglected or mistaken. One have to be very vigilant in order to act quickly by seeing your doctor for proper examination and treatment in case of any serious condition

- Digestive problems
- Chronic fatigue
- Moodiness/depression
- Food cravings
- Insulin resistance/blood sugar issues
- Rashes/skin issues
- Weight gain
- Headaches
- Allergies

Diseases Linked to Inflammation

The following are chromic health conditions associated with inflammation;

- Cancer
- Diabetes
- Cardiovascular diseases
- Pulmonary diseases
- Arithis
- Fatty liver diseases
- Alzheimer's disease
- Autoimmune diseases
- Neurological diseases

Why an Anti-Inflammatory Diet?

Eating an anti-inflammatory diet allows you to naturally reduce the level of systemic inflammation in your body through the foods you eat. There is an abundance of scientific evidence to support the healing power of healthy foods. A common element in most chronic diseases, including heart disease, diabetes, arthritis, high blood pressure, Alzheimer's disease and cancer is "chronic inflammation". This would include inflamed organs, blood vessels, brain tissue and joints. Chronic inflammation can be caused by stress, injured tissue, and by eating foods that promote inflammation or not including an abundance of anti-inflammatory foods in the diet.

Most of us have heard that abdominal fat is worse for you than hip and thigh fat. Specifically, when someone carries a lot of extra weight around their waist, a lot of it is on the inside, around our abdominal organs. These abdominal fat cells, or adipocytes, are not just sitting there being fat! They are metabolically active, especially when they are over-nourished. This can cause them to act like injured tissue, and release a lot of damaging hormones, like tumour necrosis factor, IL-6 and free radicals. These hormones can cause tissue damage elsewhere in the body, like the inside of your blood vessels, as one example. So, the anti-inflammation diet should also include increased efforts to reduce belly fat e.g. weight loss!

Some foods in particular stimulate this inflammatory reaction throughout the body. Others tend to turn the inflammation off and help repair the damage. Here are general guidelines on pro and anti-inflammatory foods:

- Damaged fats --Trans fats (hydrogenated fats) found in prepared foods & margarines (check labels), meats grilled or broiled on high heat, fried foods and refined oils.
- Fructose -- found in table sugar, high-fructose corn syrup, agave syrup, fruit juices (limit to ½ cup per day). Fruit is FINE!

- High glycemic index foods -- Foods made from flour or other ground up grains, white rice and white potatoes

Causes of Inflammation

Dietary

- Trans-fats
- Omega – 6 Fatty acids
- Refined sugars
- Gluten
- Refined grains
- Alcohol
- Food additives
- Red meat
- Dairy

Environmental factors

- Smoking or passive smoke
- Pollution
- Pesticides/herbicides
- Heavy metals

- Chemicals and airborne irritants

Stress

- Workplace
- Relationships
- Personal
- Psychological

Acute and Chronic illness

- Excess weight / obesity
- Heart disease
- Arthritis
- Celiac disease
- Crohn's disease

Genetics

- Family history

The best way to prevent or reverse systemic inflammation is to reduce exposure to the above factors. Exercising 3-5 times per week for at least 30 minutes per session will also help to reduce systemic inflammation. Another important factor to consider is stress reduction. Yoga and/or meditation which promote mental clarity can help.

Also choose to eat more anti-inflammatory foods such as:

- Blueberries
- Raw cacao
- Green tea
- Wild-caught salmon
- Ginger
- Turmeric
- Extra virgin olive oil
- Dark leafy greens
- Sweet potatoes
- Kelp

You also need to make sure you have enough Omega 3 fatty acids in your diet as they are the best anti-inflammatory drugs around. Eat oily fish such as salmon 2-3 times per week, and also supplement daily with a good quality high dose fish oil. These factors combined are all a great way to fight against silent inflammation.

Helpful hints

- Eat real foods, not too much, mostly vegetables.
- Eat fresh foods, bought recently and not left over for more than 1-2 days.
- Read the back of packaged foods – if there are more than 5 ingredients – don't eat it.
- Read the ingredients of packaged foods – if there are any numbers – don't eat it.
- Avoid white refined grains, white sugar & artificial sweeteners.
- Avoid cow's milk and cheese, instead try goats or sheep's dairy products.

- Avoid coffee and soft drinks. You really only need water, herbal teas and fresh juices.

- Make your minimal daily protein 2 portions the size of the palm of your hand (or 3 in pregnancy).

- Make sure you have protein at every meal or snack. It is the protein that fills you up and helps maintain muscle tone while losing weight.

- Use low glycemic carbohydrates where possible & only small amounts of high glycemic rice/pasta/bread as Accompaniments to, not the basis of, your meal.

- Eat frequently at least every 4-5 hours to keep blood sugar levels stable & avoid cravings. Protein providing foods keep blood sugar levels stable for longer.

- Eat your biggest meal at lunchtime rather than for dinner – or, if that's not possible make sure you have at least 2 hours between dinner and bedtime.

- Drink plenty of water (2-3 litres daily) – but remember many teas and all sweet drinks will reduce your fluid balance.

- Drinking more than one glass of water/liquid with a meal can reduce digestive activity. Avoid drinking too much water or liquid with meals.

- Fruit juice (even unsweetened) is high in sugar and low in fiber. Have a piece of fruit instead!

- Eat plenty of fibre – fruit (no more than 2-3 pieces a day), vegetables, oats, linseeds, legumes, whole grains, nuts & beans.

- Enjoy your food! And allow yourself the occasional 'treat' – then reaffirm your intentions to eat well and healthily 90% of the time.

- Replace common table salt with healthier sea salt.

- Make a delicious salad dressing to top your salad or as a dip for your steamed or baked vegetables. Choose from the following ingredients: cold pressed extra virgin olive oil, flaxseed oil, lemon juice, apple cider vinegar, wholegrain mustard, garlic, natural yoghurt, tahini & fresh herbs.

- Drink herbal teas instead of coffee or soft drink – try peppermint, chamomile, licorice, dandelion tea and green tea.

- Try some alternative milks to dairy milk – nut milks, oat milk, rice milk, coconut milk or 'Coco Quench' – a delicious combo of coconut and rick milks that are delicious in hot drinks. Homemade is best, but read the back of the packets of brought milks for the best option with the least amount of numbers.

- "The body heals 8 times faster when you exercise consistently

- Develop a morning routine: try lemon juice in warm water or Apple Cider Vinegar

- Clean out your fridge and pantry. If 'bad' foods are not in the house, then you are less likely to eat them.

- Sprinkle turmeric on your meat and/or vegetables and salad. It is a great natural anti-inflammatory.

- Eat at least 6 types of seasonal vegetables/salad every day, especially greens.

- Eat 2 serves of fresh fruit daily in a variety of colours.

- Include 2-4 serves of raw nuts, seeds and cold pressed oils in the diet everyday.

Foods that are labelled as low fat, fat free or skinny are off limits. These foods are, in fact, not healthier for you at all. The fact is that these foods have been altered away from their natural state, and usually the 'fat' that was originally present has been replace with processed sugars or carbohydrates which get absorbed and stored as fat in the body and contribute to your overall systemic inflammation. You need to give your body its best chance ever to operate at optimum health and wellness. One of the best ways to do this is to feed your body clean, natural foods that will fuel your body with vitamins, nutrient and minerals. This will not only allow your body to stay looking it's very best, but it will also keep your organs and immune system operating at their very best capacity and therefore keep you healthy on the inside as well.

The following are some of the food, ingredients or snacks to pick from;

- Steel cut or old fashioned oats or cracked grain cereal w/ toppings of your choice: chia seeds, ground flax seeds, nuts or other seeds, fresh or frozen fruit, cinnamon, coconut
- Milk (Your choice of almond, coconut, soy, etc.)
- Salad with greens (spinach, kale, romaine, etc.) leaves
- Chopped veggies: carrots, broccoli, tomato, peppers, purple onion, avocado or other veggies
- Balsamic vinaigrette dressing with 2-4 tsp. extra virgin olive oil
- Kidney beans (or other type of beans)
- Cottage cheese or chicken or seafood of choice
- Soy nuts, or other type of nut or seeds (limit to 2 Tbsp)
- Fresh Fruit
- 6 whole almonds or other nuts

- Apple or other fruit
- Salmon or other seafood or lean meat
- Sweet potato or squash
- Broccoli or other veggie
- Salad greens with chopped vegetables (carrots, tomatoes, red peppers, etc.)
- Balsamic Vinaigrette dressing (with 2 tsp. extra virgin olive oil)
- Fruit if desired

Inflammation can occur in the body as a result of a lot of things we often overlook. So, eating the right proportion and calories are key things to look out for in any case of inflammation. Below are varieties of food patients suffering from any kind of inflammation can eat. It is categorised into breakfast, lunch, dinner and snacks coupled with the ingredients and methods.

RECIPES

Breakfast

Banana Yogurt Pots

Suitable Vegetarian

Prep Time 5mins

Cook Time No cook

Serves 2

Nutrition (per serving)

- 236Kcal
- 7g   Fat
- 2g   Sat Fat
- 32g Carb
- 19g Sugar
- 4g Fibre
- 14g   Protein
- 0.1g Salt

Ingredients

- 225g / ⅞ cup Greek yogurt
- 2 bananas, sliced into chunks
- 15g / 2 tbsp walnuts, toasted and chopped

Method

1. Place some of the yogurt into the bottom of a glass. Add a layer of banana, then yogurt and repeat.
2. Once the glass is full, scatter with the nuts

Tomato & Watermelon Salad

Suitable Vegetarian

Prep Time 5mins

Cook Time No cook

Serves 2

Nutrition (per serving)

- 177 Kcal
- 13g Fat
- 5g   Sat Fat
- 13g Carb
- 10g Sugar
- 1g Fibre
- 5g   Protein
- 0.7g Salt

Ingredients

- 1 tbsp olive oil
- 1 tbsp red wine vinegar
- ¼ tsp chilli flakes
- 1 tbsp chopped mint
- 120g / ⅝ cup tomatoes, chopped
- ½ watermelon, cut into chunks
- 100g / ⅔ cup feta cheese, crumbled

Method

1. For the dressing, Mix the oil, vinegar, chilli flakes and mint and then season.
2. Put the tomatoes and watermelon into a bowl. Pour over the dressing, add the feta, and serve.

Blueberry Oats Bowl

Suitable Vegetarian

Prep Time 5mins

Cook Time 5mins

Serves 2

Nutrition (per serving)

- 235 Kcal
- 4g Fat
- 1g   Sat Fat
- 138g Carb
- 14g Sugar

- 5g Fibre
- 13g   Protein
- 0.1g Salt

Ingredients

- 60g / ⅔ cup porridge oats
- 160g / ⅗ cup Greek yogurt
- 175g / 1 ¾ cups blueberries
- 1 tsp honey

Method

1. Put the oats in a pan with 400ml of water. Heat and stir for about 2 minutes. Remove from the heat and add a third of the yogurt.
2. Tip the blueberries into a pan with the honey and 1 tbsp of water. Gently poach until the blueberries are tender.
3. Spoon the porridge into bowls and add the remaining yogurt and blueberries.

Lunch

Cannellini Bean Salad

Suitable Vegan

Prep Time 5mins

Cook Time No Cook

Serves 2

Nutrition (per serving)

- 302 Kcal
- 0g Fat
- 0g   Sat Fat
- 154g Carb
- 5g Sugar
- 25g Fibre
- 20g   Protein
- 1.2g Salt

Ingredients

- 600g / 3 cups cannellini beans

- 70g / ⅜ cup cherry tomatoes, halved
- ½ red onion, thinly sliced
- ½ tbsp red wine vinegar small bunch basil, torn

Method

1. Rinse and drain the beans and mix with the tomatoes, onion and vinegar.
2. Season, then add basil just before serving.

Edgy Veggie Wraps

Suitable Vegetarian

Prep Time 10mins

Cook Time No Cook

Serves 2

Nutrition (per serving)

- 310 Kcal
- 11g Fat
- 5g   Sat Fat
- 139g Carb
- 6g Sugar
- 8g Fibre
- 11g   Protein
- 1.6g Salt

Ingredients

- 100g / ½ cup cherry tomato
- 1 cucumber
- 6 kalamata olives
- 2 large wholemeal tortilla wraps
- 50g / ¼ cup feta cheese
- 2 tbsp hummus

Method

1. Chop the tomatoes, cut the cucumber into sticks, split the olives and remove the stones.
2. Heat the tortillas.
3. Spread the hummus over the wrap. Put the vegetable mix in the middle and roll up.

Carrot, Orange and Avocado Salad

Suitable Vegan

Prep Time 10mins

Cook Time No Cook

Serves 2

Nutrition (per serving)

- 338 Kcal
- 27g Fat
- 5g   Sat Fat

- 126g Carb
- 13g Sugar
- 11g Fibre
- 4g Protein
- 0.1g Salt

Ingredients

- 1 orange, plus zest and juice of 1
- 2 carrots, halved lengthways and sliced with a peeler
- 35g / 1 ½ cups rocket / arugula
- 1 avocado, stoned, peeled and sliced
- 1 tbsp olive oil

Method

- Cut the segments from 1 of the oranges and put in a bowl with the carrots, rocket/arugula and avocado. Whisk together the orange juice, zest and oil. Toss through the salad, and season.

Mixed Bean Salad

Suitable Vegetarian

Prep Time 10mins

Cook Time No Cook

Serves 2

Nutrition (per serving)

- 240 Kcal
- 12g Fat
- 5g   Sat Fat
- 122g Carb
- 4g Sugar
- 9g Fibre
- 11g   Protein
- 1.5g Salt

Ingredients

- 145g / ⅘ cups jar artichoke heart in oil
- ½ tbsp sundried tomato paste
- ½ tsp red wine vinegar

- 200g / 1 cup cannellini beans, drained and rinsed
- 150g / ¾ cup tomatoes, quartered handful Kalamata black olives
- 2 spring onions, thinly sliced on the diagonal
- 100g / ⅔ cups feta cheese, crumbled

Method

1. Drain the jar of artichokes, reserving 1-2 tbsp of oil. Add the oil, sun-dried tomato paste and vinegar and stir until smooth. Season to taste.

2. Chop the artichokes and tip into a bowl. Add the cannellini beans, tomatoes, olives, spring onions and half of the feta cheese. Stir in the artichoke oil mixture and tip into a serving bowl. Crumble over the remaining feta cheese, then serve.

Panzanella Salad

Suitable Vegan

Prep Time 20mins

Cook Time No Cook

Serves 2

Nutrition (per serving)

- 452 Kcal
- 35g Fat
- 6g   Sat Fat
- 137g Carb
- 7g Sugar
- 11g Fibre
- 6g   Protein
- 1.1g Salt

Ingredients

- 400g / 2 cups tomatoes
- 1 garlic clove, crushed
- 1 tbsp capers, drained and rinsed

- 1 ripe avocado, stoned, peeled and chopped
- 1 small red onion, very thinly sliced
- 2 slices of brown bread
- 2 tbsp olive oil
- 1 tbsp red wine vinegar small handful basil leaves

Method

1. Chop the tomatoes and put them in a bowl. Season well and add the garlic, capers, avocado and onion. Mix well and set aside for 10 minutes.

2. Meanwhile, tear the bread into chunks and place in a bowl. Drizzle over half of the olive oil and half of the vinegar. When ready to serve, scatter tomatoes and basil leaves and drizzle with remaining oil and vinegar. Stir before serving.

Quinoa & Stir Fry Veg

Suitable Vegan

Prep Time 15mins

Cook Time 15mins

Serves 2

Nutrition (per serving)

- 473 Kcal
- 25g Fat
- 3g   Sat Fat
- 156g Carb
- 9g Sugar
- 9g Fibre
- 11g   Protein
- 0.3g Salt

Ingredients

- 100g / ⅗ cup quinoa
- 3 tbsp olive oil
- 1 garlic clove, finely chopped

- 2 carrots, cut into thin sticks
- 150g / 1 ⅔ cups leek, sliced
- 1 broccoli head, cut into small florets
- 50g / ¼ cup tomatoes
- 100ml / ½ cup vegetable stock
- 1 tsp tomato puree juice ½ lemon

Method

1. Cook the quinoa according to pack instructions. Meanwhile, heat 3 tbsp of the oil in a pan, then add the garlic and quickly fry for 1 minute. Throw in the carrots, leeks and broccoli, then stir-fry for 2 minutes until everything is glistening.

2. Add the tomatoes, mix together the stock and tomato puree, then add to the pan. Cover and cook for 3 minutes. Drain the quinoa and toss in the remaining oil and lemon juice. Divide

between warm plates and spoon the
vegetables on top.

Moroccan Chickpea Soup

Suitable Vegan

Prep Time 5mins

Cook Time 20mins

Serves 2

Nutrition (per serving)

- 408 Kcal
- 11g Fat
- 2g   Sat Fat
- 63g Carb
- 3g Sugar
- 10g Fibre
- 15g   Protein
- 2.0g Salt

Ingredients

- 1 tbsp olive oil
- ½ medium onion, chopped
- 1 celery sticks, chopped
- 1 tsp ground cumin
- 300ml / 1 ¼ cups hot vegetable stock
- 200g can / 1 cup chopped tomatoes
- 200g can / 1 cup chickpeas, rinsed and drained
- 50g / ¼ cup frozen broad beans zest and juice ½ lemon coriander & bread to serve

Method

1. Heat the oil in a saucepan, then fry the onion and celery for 10 minutes until softened. Add the cumin and fry for another minute.

2. Turn up the heat, then add the stock, tomatoes, chickpeas and black pepper. Simmer for 8 minutes. Add broad beans

and lemon juice and cook for a further 2 minutes. Top with lemon zest and coriander.

Dinner

Moussaka

Suitable Quick

Prep Time 10mins

Cook Time 20mins

Serves 2

Nutrition (per serving)

- 577 Kcal
- 27g Fat
- 12g Sat Fat
- 46g Carb
- 6g Sugar
- 8g Fibre

- 41g Protein
- 2.8g Salt

Ingredients

- 1 tbsp olive oil
- ½ onion, finely chopped
- 1 garlic clove, finely chopped
- 250g / 9 oz lean beef mince
- 200g can / 1 cup chopped tomatoes
- 1 tbsp tomato puree
- 1 tsp ground cinnamon
- 200g / 1 cup can chickpeas
- 100g pack / ⅔ cup feta cheese, crumbled dried mint brown bread, to serve

Method

1. Heat the oil in a pan. Add the onion and garlic and fry until soft. Add the mince and fry for 3-4 minutes until browned.

2. Tip the tomatoes into the pan and stir in the tomato puree and cinnamon, then

season. Leave the mince to simmer for 20 minutes. Add the chickpeas half way through.

3. Sprinkle the feta and dried mint over the mince. Serve with toasted bread.

Spicy Tomato Baked Eggs

Suitable Quick

Prep Time 5mins

Cook Time 20mins

Serves 2

Nutrition (per serving)

- 417 Kcal
- 17g Fat
- 4g   Sat Fat
- 45g Carb
- 7g Sugar
- 5g Fibre

- 19g   Protein
- 0.8g Salt

Ingredients

- 1 tbsp olive oil
- 2 red onions, chopped
- 1 red chilli, deseeded & chopped
- 1 garlic clove, sliced small bunch coriander, stalks and leaves chopped separately
- 800g can / 4 cups cherry tomatoes
- 4 eggs
- brown bread, to serve

Method

1. Heat the oil in a frying pan with a lid, then cook the onions, chilli, garlic and coriander stalks for 5 minutes until soft. Stir in the tomatoes, then simmer for 8-10 minutes.

2. Using the back of a large spoon, make 4 dips in the sauce, then crack an egg into

each one. Put a lid on the pan, then cook over a low heat for 6-8 mins, until the eggs are done to your liking. Scatter with the coriander leaves and serve with bread.

Salmon with Potatoes and Corn Salad

Suitable Quick

Prep Time 15mins

Cook Time 15mins

Serves 2

Nutrition (per serving)

- 479 Kcal
- 21g Fat
- 3g   Sat Fat
- 27g Carb
- 2g Sugar

- 3g Fibre
- 43g   Protein
- 0.5g Salt

Ingredients

- 200g / 1 ⅓ cups baby new potatoes
- 1 sweetcorn cob
- 2 skinless salmon fillets
- 60g / ⅓ cup tomatoes

For the dressing

- 1 tbsp red wine vinegar
- 1 tbsp extra-virgin olive oil
- Bunch of spring onions/scallions, finely chopped
- 1 tbsp capers, finely chopped handful basil leaves

Method

1. Cook potatoes in boiling water until tender, adding corn for final 5 minutes. Drain & cool.

2. For the dressing, mix the vinegar, oil, spring onions / scallions, capers, basil & seasoning.

3. Heat grill to high. Rub some dressing on salmon & cook, skinned side down, for 7-8 minutes. Slice tomatoes & place on plate. Slice the potatoes, cut the corn from the cob and add to plate. Add the salmon and drizzle over the remaining dressing.

Spiced Carrot and Lentil Soup

Suitable Quick

Prep Time 10mins

Cook Time 15mins

Serves 2

Nutrition (per serving)

- 238 Kcal
- 7g Fat
- 1g   Sat Fat
- 34g Carb
- 1g Sugar
- 5g Fibre
- 11g   Protein
- 0.3g Salt

Ingredients

- 1 tsp cumin seeds pinch chilli flakes
- 1 tbsp olive oil
- 300g / 2 cups carrots, washed and coarsely grated
- 70g / ⅓ cup split red lentils
- 500ml / 2 ¼ cups hot vegetable stock
- 60ml / ¼ cup milk
- Greek yogurt, to serve

Method

1. Heat a large saucepan and dry fry the cumin seeds and chilli flakes for 1 minute. Scoop out about half of the seeds with a spoon and set aside. Add the oil, carrot, lentils, stock and milk to the pan and bring to the boil. Simmer for 15 minutes until the lentils have swollen and softened.

2. Whizz the soup with a stick blender or in a food processor until smooth. Season to taste and finish with a dollop of Greek yogurt and a sprinkling of the reserved toasted spices.

Mediterranean Chicken, Quinoa and Greek Salad

Suitable Quick

Prep Time 10mins

Cook Time 20mins

Serves 2

Nutrition (per serving)

- 424 Kcal
- 21g Fat
- 6g   Sat Fat
- 50g Carb
- 11g Sugar
- 17g Fibre
- 13g   Protein
- 1.5g Salt

Ingredients

- 100g / ⅗ cup quinoa
- ½ red chilli, deseeded and finely chopped
- 1 garlic clove, crushed
- 2 chicken breasts
- 1 tbsp extra-virgin olive oil

- 150g / ¾ cup tomatoes, roughly chopped
- handful pitted black kalamata olives
- ½ red onion, finely sliced
- 50g / ½ cup feta cheese, crumbled small bunch mint leaves, chopped juice and zest ½ lemon

Method

1. Cook the quinoa following the pack instructions, then rinse in cold water and drain thoroughly

2. Meanwhile, toss the chicken fillets in the olive oil with some seasoning, chilli and garlic. Lay in a hot pan and cook for 3-4 minutes each side or until cooked through Transfer to a plate and set aside

3. Next, tip the tomatoes, olives, onion, feta and mint into a bowl. Toss in the cooked quinoa. Stir through the

remaining olive oil, lemon juice and zest, and season well. Serve with the chicken on top.

Grilled Vegetables with Bean Mash

Suitable Vegan

Prep Time 15mins

Cook Time 25mins

Serves 2

Nutrition (per serving)

- 314 Kcal
- 16g Fat
- 2g   Sat Fat
- 33g Carb
- 9g Sugar
- 11g Fibre
- 19g Protein
- 0.1g Salt

Ingredients

- 1 pepper, deseeded & quartered
- 1 aubergine, sliced lengthways
- 2 courgettes, sliced lengthways
- 2 tbsp olive oil
- For the mash
- 400g can / 2 cups haricot beans, rinsed
- 1 garlic clove, crushed
- 100ml / ½ cup vegetable stock
- 1 tbsp chopped coriander

Method

1. Heat the grill. Arrange the vegetables over a grill pan &brush lightly with oil. Grill until lightly browned, turn them over, brush again with oil, then grill until tender.

2. Meanwhile, put the beans in a pan with garlic and stock. Bring to the boil, then simmer, uncovered, for 10 minutes. Mash roughly with a potato masher.

Divide the vegetables and mash between 2 plates, drizzle over oil & sprinkle with black pepper and coriander.

Spicy Mediterranean Beet Salad

Prep Time 10mins

Cook Time 30mins

Serves 2

Nutrition (per serving)

- 548 Kcal
- 20g Fat
- 4g   Sat Fat
- 58g Carb
- 6g Sugar
- 11g Fibre
- 23g   Protein
- 1.7g Salt

Ingredients

- 8 raw baby beetroots, or 4 medium, scrubbed
- ½ tbsp sumac
- ½ tbsp ground cumin
- 400g can / 2 cups chickpeas, drained and rinsed
- 2 tbsp olive oil
- ½ tsp lemon zest
- ½ tsp lemon juice
- 200g / ½ cup Greek yogurt
- 1 tbsp harissa paste
- 1 tsp crushed red chilli flakes
- mint leaves, chopped, to serve

Method

1. Heat oven to 425F/220C/200C fan/gas 7. Halve or quarter beetroots depending on size. Mix spices together. On a large baking tray, mix chickpeas and beetroot with the oil. Season with salt & sprinkle

over the spices. Mix again. Roast for 30 minutes.

2. While the vegetables are cooking, mix the lemon zest and juice with the yogurt. Swirl the harissa through and spread into a bowl. Top with the beetroot & chickpeas, and sprinkle with the chilli flakes & mint.

Snacks

Strawberry and Yogurt Parfait

Prep Time 5mins

Cook Time 0min

Serves 2

Nutrition (per serving)

- 161Kcal

- 4g Fat

- 1g Sat Fat

- 23g Carb
- 13g Sugar
- 2g Fibre
- 9g   Protein
- 0.1g Salt

Ingredients

- 150g / ¾ cup punnet strawberries, chopped
- 1 tbsp sugar
- 150g / ½ cup Greek yogurt
- 4 small amaretti biscuit, crushed

Method

1. · In a small bowl, mix the strawberries with half the sugar, then roughly mash them with a fork.
2. Mix the remaining sugar into the yogurt, then layer up 6 glasses with amaretti biscuits, yogurt and strawberries.

Mediterranean Dip

Suitable Vegetarian

Prep Time 10mins

Cook Time 0min

Serves 4

Nutrition (per serving)

- 213 Kcal
- 12g Fat
- 7g   Sat Fat
- 16g Carb
- 2g Sugar
- 4g Fibre
- 10g   Protein
- 1.5g Salt

Ingredients

- 400g can / 2 cups cannellini bean
- 200g / ⅞ cups feta cheese
- 1 tbsp lemon juice

- 1 garlic clove, crushed
- 3 tbsp chopped dill, mint or chives
- (or 1 tbsp each)

Method

1. Drain and rinse beans. Tip into a food processor with feta, lemon juice and garlic. Whizz until smooth.
2. Add dill, mint or chives, and season with pepper.

Honeyed Figs with Yogurt and Almonds

Suitable Vegetarian

Prep Time 5mins

Cook Time 0min

Serves 1

Nutrition (per serving)

- 151 Kcal
- 5g Fat
- 1g   Sat Fat
- 24g Carb
- 11g Sugar
- 2g Fibre
- 4g   Protein
- 0.1g Salt

Ingredients

- 2 figs
- 2 tbsp Greek yogurt
- 1 tbsp honey
- 2 pinches of cinnamon
- handful flaked toasted almonds

Method

1. Cut the figs in half. Spoon over the yogurt, then drizzle with honey.

2. Sprinkle with cinnamon and a few flaked
toasted almonds.

Physical Activities and Stress Management in the cases of Inflammation

The importance of exercise and rest to the body system cannot be overemphasised. Exercise and rest according to research are one of the doctors of the body system. When we eat the right proportion and proper calories of food, exercise regularly and have adequate rest, the body can heal from diseases even without any sort of drugs prescribed by a medical practitioner. The following are tips to follow to;

- Physical activity, yoga, meditation, and other mindful movement promote peace and balance in the nervous system, counteracting the damage of psychological stress.

- A good night's sleep (at least 7-9 hours) decreases inflammatory chemicals in the body and allows for self-repair.
- Nourish your body regularly with non-food pleasures which create endorphins for powerful healing: dancing, hot baths, massage, sex, laughter: whatever makes you feel really good.
- Remember that some stress can be a powerful motivator and allow you to create change in the world. Embrace necessary stress and let yourself find peace within chaos.